SLEEPLESS IN THE NEW NORMAL

The Ultimate Guide to Reclaiming Your Sleep and Dreams post COVID

Thomas Murray

Table of Contents

Chapter 1: Introduction

The COVID-19 pandemic has been an unprecedented event that has impacted our daily lives in countless ways. One area that has been significantly affected is our sleep and dreams. With the pandemic forcing many of us to stay indoors and disrupting our daily routines, our sleep schedules and dream patterns had been thrown out of whack. The disruption led to many of us being sleepless and an increase in sleep problems including insomnia and nightmares, and has left many of us feeling tired and groggy during the day. For many of us, the same problems continue even when the pandemic abated.

In this book, we aim to help you reclaim your sleep and dreams post COVID by providing you with the tools and strategies you need to improve your sleep quality and quantity, and enhance your dream experiences. We believe that sleep and dreams are essential for overall health and well-being, and that getting a good night's sleep and having meaningful dream experiences can make all the difference in our lives.

We'll start by discussing the importance of sleep and dreams for physical and mental health. We'll explore the many ways in which poor sleep can impact our health, from increasing our risk of chronic diseases to impairing our cognitive functioning. We'll also dive into the fascinating world of dreams and discuss the many benefits they can provide, from improving our problem-solving abilities to facilitating emotional healing.

We'll then move on to discuss the impact of COVID-19 on sleep and dreams. We'll explore the various ways in which the pandemic has disrupted our sleep patterns and dream experiences, and the many challenges that have arisen as a result. From the stress and anxiety caused by the pandemic to the changes in our daily routines, there are also many factors that have contributed to the disruption of our sleep and dreams.

The next section of the book will focus on practical strategies and techniques for improving sleep quality and quantity, and enhancing dream experiences. We'll discuss the importance of establishing a regular sleep routine, creating a relaxing sleep environment, and practicing good sleep hygiene. We'll also explore the many ways in which technology can be used to promote healthy sleep and enhance dream experiences.

Finally, we'll take a look at the future of sleep and dream science, and the many exciting developments that are on the horizon. From new technologies for monitoring and analyzing sleep and dreams to the development of new treatments for sleep disorders, the future of sleep and dream science is filled with promise.

We hope that this book will provide you with the knowledge and tools you need to improve your sleep and dreams post COVID. Whether you're struggling with insomnia, nightmares, or other sleep problems, we believe that the strategies and techniques outlined in this book will help you get the restful sleep you need and deserve. So, let's get started and get you on the path to better sleep and dream experiences.

Chapter 2: Understanding Sleep

Sleep is an essential part of our lives, and it's something that we spend a third of our time doing. It's a complex and fascinating phenomenon that scientists are still studying to this day. In this chapter, we'll dive into the science of sleep and explore the different stages of sleep, the benefits of sleep, and the factors that can impact our sleep.

The Stages of Sleep

Sleep is divided into two main categories: non-REM (rapid eye movement) sleep and REM sleep. Non-REM sleep is further divided into three stages, while REM sleep is its own distinct stage.

Stage 1: This is the lightest stage of sleep and typically lasts for only a few minutes. During this stage, your heart rate and breathing slow down, and your muscles begin to relax. It's common to experience sudden muscle contractions or a feeling of falling during this stage.

Stage 2: This is a deeper stage of sleep that makes up the majority of our sleep time. During this stage, our brain waves slow down, and our body temperature drops. This is also the stage where we experience sleep spindles and Kcomplexes, which are brief bursts of brain activity that help us maintain sleep.

Stage 3: This is the deepest stage of sleep, also known as slow-wave sleep. During this stage, our brain waves slow down even further, and it becomes difficult to awaken us. This is the stage of sleep where we experience the most physical restoration, and it's essential for the body to repair and rejuvenate itself.

REM Sleep: REM sleep is the stage of sleep where we experience the most vivid and memorable dreams. During this stage, our brain waves become more active, and our breathing and heart rate increase. Our muscles become paralyzed to prevent us from acting out our dreams.

The Benefits of Sleep

Getting enough sleep is critical for good health and well-being. It's during sleep that our bodies repair and restore themselves, and our brains consolidate memories and process emotions. Here are some of the benefits of getting enough sleep:

Improved physical health: Getting enough sleep can reduce the risk of chronic diseases such as diabetes, heart disease, and obesity.

Better cognitive functioning: Sleep is essential for good cognitive functioning, including memory, attention, and decision-making.

Emotional regulation: Sleep is critical for emotional regulation and can help us better manage stress and anxiety.

Enhanced athletic performance: Getting enough sleep can improve athletic performance by reducing fatigue and enhancing physical recovery.

Factors That Impact Sleep

Several factors can impact our sleep, including our environment, lifestyle, and physical health.

Environment: The environment we sleep in can have a significant impact on our sleep quality. A quiet, dark, and cool room is ideal for sleep, while noise, light, and temperature can all disrupt sleep.

Lifestyle: Our lifestyle choices can also impact our sleep quality. Drinking alcohol or caffeine, eating heavy meals, and not exercising regularly can all interfere with sleep. It's essential to establish healthy sleep habits and create a relaxing sleep environment.

Physical Health: Several physical health conditions can impact sleep, including sleep apnea, restless legs syndrome, and chronic pain. It's essential to seek medical advice if you're experiencing ongoing sleep problems.

Sleep is a fascinating and essential part of our lives, and understanding the science of sleep can help us better appreciate its importance. By improving our sleep habits, creating a relaxing sleep environment, and seeking medical advice when necessary, we can enjoy the many benefits of a good night's sleep.

Chapter 3: Sleep Deprivation and its Consequences

Sleep deprivation is a widespread problem in modern society. With the demands of work, family, and social life, it's easy to sacrifice sleep to get more done. However, chronic sleep deprivation can have severe consequences on our physical and mental health. In this chapter, we'll explore the consequences of sleep deprivation, including some unconventional ideas for addressing the issue.

Consequences of Sleep Deprivation

Lack of sleep affects the body in several ways, including:

Impaired cognitive function: Sleep deprivation can affect cognitive function, including memory, attention, and decision-making. Inadequate sleep can also affect creativity and problem-solving abilities.

Increased risk of accidents: Sleep-deprived individuals are more likely to have accidents, both on the road and in the workplace.

Reduced immune system function: Chronic sleep deprivation can weaken the immune system, making individuals more susceptible to illness.

Increased risk of chronic diseases: Sleep deprivation is linked to several chronic diseases, including diabetes, heart disease, and obesity.

Mood disturbances: Sleep deprivation can lead to irritability, mood swings, and depression.

Unconventional Ideas for Addressing Sleep Deprivation

Nap rooms in the workplace: Many companies are now recognizing the importance of sleep and are providing nap rooms for employees to take a quick nap during the workday. A short nap of 20-30 minutes can help to improve cognitive function and reduce fatigue.

"Sleep bars": Similar to coffee shops, sleep bars are a new trend that allows individuals to pay for a private space to take a nap or relax during the day. These sleep bars provide a quiet, dark environment that can promote relaxation and rest.

"Digital sunset" routines: The blue light emitted by electronic devices can interfere with sleep. One way to address this issue is to establish a "digital sunset" routine where electronic devices are turned off or put away at a specific time before bedtime.

Mindful breathing: Mindful breathing is a technique that involves taking deep, slow breaths to promote relaxation and reduce stress. Incorporating this technique into a bedtime routine can help to calm the mind and promote better sleep.

Music therapy: Listening to calming music before bed can help to promote relaxation and reduce stress. Some studies suggest that music can improve sleep quality, particularly in individuals who have difficulty falling asleep.

Acupuncture: Acupuncture is a traditional Chinese medicine technique that involves inserting needles into specific points on the body. Some studies suggest that acupuncture can improve sleep quality and reduce insomnia.

Overall, sleep deprivation is a prevalent problem that can have severe consequences on our physical and mental health. While there are several conventional methods for addressing sleep deprivation, including establishing a regular sleep routine and creating a sleep-conducive environment, there are also some unconventional ideas that can be effective. By incorporating some of these ideas into our daily routine, we can improve our sleep quality and promote better overall health and well-being. In the next chapter, we'll explore the fascinating world of dreams and their potential to improve our lives.

Chapter 4: Dreams and their Significance

Dreams have fascinated humans for thousands of years. Ancient civilizations believed that dreams held significant meaning and provided insight into the future. Today, while the interpretation of dreams is still a topic of debate, researchers have discovered that dreams can provide valuable insights into our emotional and mental state. In this chapter, we'll explore the significance of dreams and how they can impact our waking life.

The Purpose of Dreams

While the exact purpose of dreams is still unknown, researchers have discovered some potential reasons for why we dream. Some theories suggest that dreams serve to help us process emotions and memories, while others believe that they are a byproduct of the brain's activities during sleep. Regardless of their purpose, dreams provide a unique window into our subconscious mind and can provide valuable insights into our emotional state.

The Significance of Dreams

Dreams can provide insight into our emotional and mental state, including our fears, desires, and anxieties. By analyzing our dreams, we can gain a better understanding of our innermost thoughts and feelings. Dreams can also be a source of creativity and inspiration, as they can provide new perspectives and ideas.

Types of Dreams

There are several different types

of dreams, each with its unique characteristics and significance. Some of the most common types of dreams include:

Lucid Dreams: Lucid dreams occur when the dreamer becomes aware that they are dreaming. In a lucid dream, the dreamer can often control the dream's outcome, which can be a valuable tool for overcoming fears or achieving goals.

Recurring Dreams: Recurring dreams are dreams that happen repeatedly over an extended period. These dreams may indicate unresolved issues or concerns that need to be addressed.

Nightmares: Nightmares are dreams that cause the dreamer to wake up feeling scared or anxious. These dreams may be a manifestation of unresolved fears or past trauma.

Daydreams: Daydreams are not necessarily a type of dream that occurs during sleep, but rather a form of spontaneous imagination that occurs while awake. Daydreaming can be a valuable tool for creativity and problem-solving.

Interpreting Dreams

The interpretation of dreams has been a topic of debate for centuries. Some believe that dreams have a symbolic meaning that can be interpreted to provide insight into our lives. Others believe that dreams are a random sequence of thoughts that have no inherent meaning. While the interpretation of dreams remains subjective, many believe that dreams can provide valuable insights into our subconscious mind and emotional state.

Tools for Understanding Dreams

Several tools can be used to help understand the significance of dreams, including:

Dream Journals: Keeping a dream journal is a valuable tool for understanding the recurring themes and symbols in our dreams. By recording our dreams regularly, we can begin to identify patterns and gain a better understanding of our subconscious mind.

Dream Analysis: Dream analysis is a technique used to interpret the symbolism and meaning of dreams. A trained therapist or counselor can help to identify the themes and symbols in our dreams and provide insights into our emotional and mental state.

Meditation and Visualization: Meditation and visualization can be valuable tools for understanding our dreams. By meditating on the symbols and themes in our dreams, we can gain a deeper understanding of our innermost thoughts and emotions.

Dreams are a fascinating and complex phenomenon that can provide valuable insights into our emotional and mental state. While the interpretation of dreams remains subjective, the significance of dreams is undeniable. By exploring our dreams and analyzing their symbolism and themes, we can gain a better understanding of our innermost thoughts and feelings. In the next chapter, we'll explore some practical tips and strategies for improving the quality of our sleep and promoting healthy dreams.

Chapter 5: The Impact of Stress on Sleep and Dreams

Stress is a common experience in today's fast-paced world. The COVID-19 pandemic has only heightened the levels of stress experienced by many people. Stress can have a significant impact on our physical and mental health, including our sleep and dreams. In this chapter, we'll explore the impact of stress on sleep and dreams and discuss strategies for managing stress to promote healthy sleep and dreams.

The Physiology of Stress

Stress is a natural response to perceived threats, and it triggers a physiological response known as the "fight or flight" response. When we experience stress, our bodies release cortisol, adrenaline, and other stress hormones, which can lead to physical and emotional changes. These changes can include increased heart rate, rapid breathing, and heightened alertness.

The Impact of Stress on Sleep

Stress can have a significant impact on our ability to sleep. The release of stress hormones can lead to difficulty falling asleep or staying asleep. Stress can also cause nightmares, vivid dreams, and frequent waking during the night. Chronic stress can lead to insomnia, a sleep disorder that causes difficulty falling asleep, staying asleep, or both.

The Impact of Stress on Dreams

Stress can also impact our dreams. When we experience stress during the day, it can manifest in our dreams as nightmares or vivid, intense dreams. Chronic stress can lead to recurrent nightmares, which can significantly impact our quality of life. Stress can also cause us to remember our dreams more vividly, leading to more intense emotional experiences.

Strategies for Managing Stress

Managing stress is essential for promoting healthy sleep and dreams. Some strategies for managing stress include:

Mindfulness and Meditation: Mindfulness and meditation are techniques that can help to reduce stress and promote relaxation. By focusing on the present moment and our breathing, we can reduce the impact of stress on our bodies and minds.

Exercise: Exercise is a natural stress reliever that can help to promote healthy sleep and reduce the impact of stress on our dreams.

Sleep Hygiene: Practicing good sleep hygiene, such as creating a relaxing sleep environment, avoiding screens before bedtime, and sticking to a regular sleep schedule, can help to reduce the impact of stress on our sleep and dreams.

Cognitive Behavioral Therapy: Cognitive-behavioral therapy is a type of therapy that can help to reduce the impact of stress on our sleep and dreams. This type of therapy focuses on changing negative thought patterns and behaviors that may be contributing to stress and sleep problems.

Stress can significantly impact our sleep and dreams. By understanding the physiology of stress and its impact on our bodies and minds, we can take steps to manage stress and promote healthy sleep and dreams. Mindfulness, exercise, good sleep hygiene, and cognitive-behavioral therapy are all effective strategies for reducing the impact of stress on our sleep and dreams. In the next chapter, we'll explore the role of diet and nutrition in promoting healthy sleep and dreams.

Chapter 6: How Technology Affects Sleep and Dreams

In today's digital age, we are more connected than ever before. The prevalence of technology has made our lives more convenient, efficient, and entertaining. However, this constant connection can come at a cost, particularly when it comes to our sleep and dreams. The impact of technology on our sleep and dreams is a growing concern, and in this chapter, we'll explore this topic in detail.

The Impact of Technology on Sleep

The blue light emitted by electronic devices such as smartphones, tablets, and computers can suppress the production of melatonin, the hormone that regulates our sleep-wake cycle. Exposure to blue light before bedtime can disrupt our natural sleep patterns and lead to difficulty falling asleep and staying asleep. Studies have found that the use of electronic devices before bedtime is associated with poor sleep quality, insomnia, and sleep disorders.

In addition to the impact of blue light, technology can also disrupt our sleep by increasing our level of alertness. The use of electronic devices such as smartphones and tablets can stimulate our brains and make it difficult for us to unwind and relax before bedtime. The constant stimulation of our brains can lead to increased stress, anxiety, and difficulty falling asleep.

The Impact of Technology on Dreams

While the impact of technology on our sleep is clear, its impact on our dreams is less understood. However, there is evidence to suggest that technology can influence the content and vividness of our dreams. Watching violent or disturbing content before bed can lead to nightmares or more vivid dreams. In addition, the use of technology in bed can lead to a state of hyperarousal, which can make it more difficult to fall asleep and lead to less restful sleep.

The Impact of Social Media on Sleep and Dreams

Social media has become an integral part of our lives, but it can also have a negative impact on our sleep and dreams. The constant stream of information and notifications can make it difficult to disconnect and relax before bedtime. In addition, the fear of missing out (FOMO) can cause anxiety and stress, leading to poor sleep quality.

Strategies for Managing Technology Use

While it may not be possible to completely eliminate technology from our lives, there are strategies we can use to manage its impact on our sleep and dreams. Here are some of the most effective strategies:

Limit screen time before bed: Avoiding the use of electronic devices before bedtime can help your body wind down and prepare for sleep. Try to avoid using electronic devices for at least an hour before bedtime to give your body time to produce melatonin and prepare for sleep.

Use blue light filters: Many devices now have a blue light filter or night mode that reduces the amount of blue light emitted. Using these features can help reduce the impact of blue light on your sleep.

Create a technology-free bedroom: Make your bedroom a technology-free zone by removing all electronic devices from your sleeping area. This will help you associate your bedroom with sleep and relaxation rather than work and stimulation.

Avoid social media before bed: Try to avoid using social media before bed to reduce the risk of FOMO and the anxiety it can cause. Instead, consider reading a book or practicing relaxation techniques to help you unwind.

Use technology to enhance sleep: While technology can disrupt our sleep, it can also be used to enhance it. Sleep-tracking apps and smartwatches can provide insights into our sleep patterns and help us make positive changes to our sleep habits.

Overall, technology has become an integral part of our lives, and while it offers many benefits, its impact on our sleep and dreams cannot be ignored. By understanding the impact of technology on our sleep and dreams, we can take steps to manage its influence and ensure that we get the restful sleep we need for our physical and mental well-being.

Chapter 7: Sleep Disorders

Sleep disorders are conditions that affect a person's ability to get a restful night's sleep. These disorders can be caused by a variety of factors, such as genetics, lifestyle, or medical conditions, and can have a significant impact on a person's overall health and well-being. In this chapter, we will explore the most common sleep disorders, their causes, and effective treatment options.

Insomnia

Insomnia is the most common sleep disorder, affecting up to one-third of the adult population. It is characterized by difficulty falling or staying asleep and can be caused by a variety of factors, including stress, anxiety, depression, and certain medications. Insomnia can have a significant impact on a person's mental and physical health, leading to daytime fatigue, irritability, and difficulty concentrating.

There are several effective treatments for insomnia, including cognitive-behavioral therapy (CBT), which helps to identify and change negative thought patterns and behaviors that contribute to sleep difficulties. Medications such as benzodiazepines and non-benzodiazepine sedatives can also be effective in treating insomnia, but they should only be used under the guidance of a medical professional.

Sleep Apnea

Sleep apnea is a serious sleep disorder that affects an estimated 22 million Americans. It is characterized by pauses in breathing during sleep, which can lead to daytime fatigue, headaches, and irritability. Sleep apnea is often caused by an obstruction in the airway, such as the tongue or soft tissue in the back of the throat, and can lead to long-term health problems if left untreated.

One of the most effective treatments for sleep apnea is continuous positive airway pressure (CPAP) therapy. This treatment involves wearing a mask over the nose and/or mouth that delivers a steady stream of air to keep the airway open during sleep. Other treatments for sleep apnea include lifestyle changes, such as weight loss, and surgery to remove obstructions in the airway.

Restless Leg Syndrome

Restless leg syndrome (RLS) is a neurological disorder that affects up to 10% of the population. It is characterized by an irresistible urge to move the legs, particularly at night, which can disrupt sleep and lead to daytime fatigue. RLS is often caused by an imbalance of dopamine, a neurotransmitter that helps to regulate movement, and can be worsened by certain medications or medical conditions.

There are several effective treatments for RLS, including medications that increase dopamine levels, such as dopamine agonists and levodopa. Lifestyle changes, such as avoiding caffeine and alcohol, and regular exercise, can also help to reduce the symptoms of RLS.

Narcolepsy

Narcolepsy is a rare neurological disorder that affects an estimated 1 in 2,000 people. It is characterized by excessive daytime sleepiness, sudden and uncontrollable bouts of sleep, and often accompanied by cataplexy, a sudden loss of muscle tone triggered by strong emotions such as laughter or surprise. Narcolepsy is caused by a lack of hypocretin, a neurotransmitter that helps to regulate wakefulness and REM sleep.

There is no cure for narcolepsy, but several treatments can help to manage its symptoms. Medications such as stimulants and antidepressants can help to reduce excessive daytime sleepiness, while sodium oxybate can help to improve nighttime sleep and reduce the frequency of cataplexy episodes. Lifestyle changes, such as maintaining a regular sleep schedule and avoiding alcohol and caffeine, can also be effective in managing narcolepsy.

Parasomnias

Parasomnias are a group of sleep disorders that involve abnormal behavior or experiences during sleep, such as sleepwalking, sleep talking, and night terrors. These disorders can be caused by a variety of factors, such as genetics, stress, or medical conditions, and can have a significant impact on a person's mental and physical health.

Treatment for parasomnias often involves identifying and addressing the underlying cause of the disorder. In some cases, medications such as benzodiazepines can be effective in reducing the frequency and severity of parasomnia episodes. Other treatments, such as relaxation techniques and maintaining a regular sleep schedule, can also be helpful in managing parasomnias.

Sleep disorders can have a significant impact on a person's quality of life, affecting their mental and physical health, and productivity. It is essential to identify and address these disorders to ensure that individuals can get the restful, restorative sleep they need. By understanding the common sleep disorders, their causes, and effective treatment options, individuals can take steps to improve their sleep and overall well-being. It is important to consult a medical professional if sleep difficulties persist, as they can help to identify underlying medical conditions or recommend appropriate treatment options.

Chapter 8: The Importance of Circadian Rhythms

Circadian rhythms are the natural, internal 24-hour cycles that regulate the sleep-wake cycle, as well as other bodily functions, such as hormone production, digestion, and body temperature. These rhythms are controlled by a complex system of biological clocks in the brain and throughout the body, which respond to cues such as light and darkness.

The Importance of Circadian Rhythms

Circadian rhythms play a crucial role in regulating many of the body's physiological processes, and disruptions to these rhythms can have significant health implications. Research has shown that circadian rhythm disruptions have been linked to an increased risk of obesity, diabetes, cardiovascular disease, and other health conditions.

Disruptions to circadian rhythms can also have a significant impact on sleep quality and quantity. For example, exposure to artificial light, particularly blue light emitted by electronic devices, can disrupt the natural sleep-wake cycle by suppressing the production of melatonin, a hormone that helps to regulate sleep. This disruption can result in difficulty falling asleep, waking up during the night, and feeling groggy and fatigued during the day.

Practical Tips for Supporting Circadian Rhythms

There are several practical steps that individuals can take to support their circadian rhythms and improve their overall health and well-being. These include:

Regulating exposure to light: Exposure to natural light during the day can help to regulate the sleep-wake cycle and support healthy circadian rhythms. Conversely, avoiding exposure to artificial light, particularly in the hours leading up to bedtime, can help to promote better sleep and reduce the risk of circadian rhythm disruptions.

Maintaining a regular sleep schedule: Going to bed and waking up at the same time each day can help to support healthy circadian rhythms and improve sleep quality and quantity.

Avoiding caffeine and alcohol: Caffeine and alcohol can disrupt the sleep-wake cycle and negatively impact circadian rhythms. Limiting consumption of these substances can help to promote healthy circadian rhythms and improve sleep quality.

Creating a sleep-friendly environment: A dark, quiet, and cool bedroom can help to support healthy sleep and promote circadian rhythms. Installing blackout curtains

or blinds can help to reduce exposure to outside light, while keeping the room cool and using white noise machines or earplugs can help to block out noise.

Using technology to support circadian rhythms: There are several apps and devices available that can help to support healthy circadian rhythms. These include blue light blocking glasses, which can be worn in the evening to reduce exposure to artificial light, and smart light bulbs that can be programmed to adjust the color and intensity of light according to the time of day.

Circadian rhythms are a fundamental aspect of our physiology, and disruptions to these rhythms can have significant health implications, particularly with regards to sleep quality and quantity. By adopting practical steps to support healthy circadian rhythms, individuals can improve their sleep and overall health and well-being.

Chapter 9: The Role of Nutrition in Sleep

While many people focus on external factors like light, noise, and stress when it comes to improving their sleep, one important factor that is often overlooked is nutrition. What we eat and drink can have a significant impact on the quality and duration of our sleep, as well as our overall health and well-being. In this chapter, we will explore the role of nutrition in sleep and provide practical tips for improving your sleep through your diet.

The Link Between Nutrition and Sleep

There is a complex interplay between diet and sleep, with both influencing each other in various ways. Studies have shown that nutrient deficiencies can lead to sleep disturbances, and that poor sleep quality can impact our appetite, food choices, and metabolism. For example, individuals who sleep less than seven hours per night have been found to be more likely to consume high calorie, high fat, and high sugar foods than those who sleep for a longer duration.

On the other hand, consuming certain nutrients can have a positive impact on sleep. For example, consuming foods rich in tryptophan, an amino acid that is a precursor to the sleep-inducing hormone melatonin, can help to promote healthy sleep. Foods that are high in magnesium, such as leafy greens, nuts, and whole grains, have also been shown to be beneficial for sleep.

Practical Tips for Improving Sleep Through Nutrition

There are several practical steps that individuals can take to improve their sleep through their diet. These include:

Avoiding caffeine and alcohol: Caffeine and alcohol can both have a negative impact on sleep quality and duration. It is recommended to avoid consuming caffeine after midday and to limit alcohol consumption, particularly in the hours leading up to bedtime.

Consuming foods rich in tryptophan: Tryptophan is an amino acid that is essential for the production of melatonin, which plays a crucial role in regulating the sleep-wake cycle. Foods that are high in tryptophan include turkey, chicken, fish, eggs, nuts, and seeds.

Incorporating foods rich in magnesium: Magnesium is a mineral that has been shown to be beneficial for sleep, as it helps to relax muscles and reduce stress.

Foods that are high in magnesium include leafy greens, nuts, seeds, whole grains, and legumes.

Consuming foods rich in vitamin B6: Vitamin B6 is an important nutrient for the production of melatonin. Foods that are high in vitamin B6 include fish, poultry, bananas, nuts, and seeds.

Avoiding large meals before bedtime: Consuming a large meal before bedtime can make it difficult to fall asleep and can result in digestive issues. It is recommended to finish eating at least two to three hours before bedtime.

Nutrition plays a critical role in regulating sleep, and making dietary changes can have a positive impact on sleep quality and duration. By incorporating foods that are rich in sleep-promoting nutrients and avoiding foods and drinks that can disrupt sleep, individuals can improve their overall sleep and promote better health and well-being.

Chapter 10: The Benefits of Exercise for Sleep and Dreams

While it is widely known that exercise is beneficial for physical health, many people may not realize the significant impact it can have on sleep and dreams. In this chapter, we will explore the benefits of exercise for sleep and dreams and provide practical tips for incorporating physical activity into your daily routine.

The Link Between Exercise and Sleep

Research has shown that regular exercise can lead to improved sleep quality, as well as increased duration of sleep. Exercise has been found to increase the amount of deep sleep and REM sleep, the two most important stages of the sleep cycle for physical and mental restoration. Additionally, individuals who exercise regularly have been found to have less trouble falling asleep and staying asleep, as well as a reduced likelihood of experiencing sleep disorders.

The mechanisms behind the positive effects of exercise on sleep are not yet fully understood, but several theories have been proposed. One theory suggests that exercise increases the production of endorphins, which are chemicals that can induce feelings of relaxation and well-being, and can help to counteract the negative effects of stress on sleep. Another theory suggests that exercise may help to regulate the body's circadian rhythm, the internal clock that regulates the sleep-wake cycle.

The Link Between Exercise and Dreams

Exercise has also been found to have a positive impact on dreams. Studies have shown that individuals who exercise regularly report having more positive, vivid, and memorable dreams than those who are more sedentary. Additionally, exercise has been found to be beneficial for individuals who suffer from nightmare disorder, a condition in which individuals experience frequent and distressing nightmares.

The mechanisms behind the positive effects of exercise on dreams are not yet fully understood, but several theories have been proposed. One theory suggests that exercise may help to regulate the brain's neurotransmitters, the chemicals that help to facilitate communication between nerve cells, and can help to promote more positive and less disturbing dream content. Another theory suggests that exercise may help to reduce stress and anxiety, which can lead to more positive and less disturbing dreams.

Practical Tips for Incorporating Exercise into Your Daily Routine

In order to reap the benefits of exercise for sleep and dreams, it is important to incorporate physical activity into your daily routine. Here are some practical tips for doing so:

Set realistic goals: Start by setting realistic goals for yourself, and gradually increase the intensity and duration of your workouts as you become more comfortable.

Choose activities you enjoy: Exercise doesn't have to mean running on a treadmill or lifting weights at the gym. Find activities that you enjoy, such as dancing, swimming, or hiking, and make them a regular part of your routine.

Time your workouts strategically: While exercise is beneficial for sleep and dreams, it is important to time your workouts strategically. Avoid exercising too close to bedtime, as this can make it difficult to fall asleep.

Make exercise a social activity: Consider working out with a friend or joining a sports team or fitness class. This can help to keep you motivated and make exercise more enjoyable.

Incorporate mindfulness and relaxation techniques: Consider incorporating mindfulness and relaxation techniques into your exercise routine, such as yoga or tai chi. These activities can help to reduce stress and promote relaxation, which can be beneficial for sleep and dreams.

Exercise is a powerful tool for improving sleep and dreams, and incorporating physical activity into your daily routine can have a significant positive impact on your overall health and well-being. By setting realistic goals, choosing activities you enjoy, timing your workouts strategically, making exercise a social activity, and incorporating mindfulness and relaxation techniques, you can make exercise a regular part of your routine and reap the benefits for sleep and dreams.

Chapter 11: How to Create the Ideal Sleep Environment

The environment in which you sleep can play a significant role in the quality of your sleep. Creating the ideal sleep environment can lead to a better night's rest, helping you to feel refreshed and energized in the morning. In this chapter, we will explore the various elements that make up the perfect sleep environment, including lighting, noise, temperature, and comfort.

Lighting:

The lighting in your sleep environment can significantly impact your body's natural circadian rhythm. The circadian rhythm is your body's internal 24-hour clock that regulates your sleep-wake cycle. Exposure to bright light in the morning and avoiding bright light in the evening can help to regulate your circadian rhythm.

In the evening, dimming the lights can help your body to prepare for sleep. This can be achieved by using soft yellow light or warm white bulbs. Avoid bright blue light, such as the light emitted by electronic devices like phones and tablets, as this can suppress the release of the sleep hormone, melatonin.

In the morning, exposing yourself to bright light can help to reset your body's internal clock. You can achieve this by opening your curtains to let in natural light, using a light therapy lamp, or going for a walk outside.

Noise:

Noise can be a significant disturbance to your sleep environment. Loud noises can disrupt your sleep, causing you to wake up, and reducing the quality of your sleep. Even if you don't fully wake up, noise can disturb your sleep cycle, causing you to spend less time in the deeper, restorative stages of sleep.

To reduce the impact of noise on your sleep, use earplugs, noise-canceling headphones, or a white noise machine. White noise machines produce a constant, soothing sound that can help to mask background noise, allowing you to fall asleep and stay asleep.

Temperature:

The temperature of your sleep environment can significantly affect your sleep quality. Your body temperature naturally drops as you fall asleep, and a cooler sleep environment can help to facilitate this. A room temperature of around 18-20 degrees Celsius is considered ideal for sleep.

It's essential to choose the right bedding to help regulate your body temperature during the night. Breathable fabrics such as cotton, bamboo, or linen can help to prevent overheating, while flannel and fleece are best reserved for colder months.

Comfort:

The comfort of your bed is essential for getting a good night's sleep. A good mattress, pillow, and bedding are all essential elements in creating the perfect sleep environment.

A comfortable mattress should provide the right level of support for your body, and your pillow should be the correct height to keep your head and neck in a neutral position. Your bedding should be soft and cozy, creating a comfortable and welcoming environment for sleep.

Additional tips for creating the ideal sleep environment:

1.Use blackout curtains to block out light and keep your room dark while you sleep.

2.Keep your bedroom clean and tidy to create a relaxing and peaceful environment.

3.Reserve your bed for sleep and intimacy only, avoiding using it for work or leisure activities.

4.Avoid using electronic devices in your bed as the blue light they emit can interfere with your sleep.

5.If you have a pet that sleeps in your bed, consider providing them with their own sleeping space.

Creating the ideal sleep environment can go a long way in helping you to achieve a better night's sleep. By paying attention to the lighting, noise, temperature, and comfort of your sleep environment, you can create a relaxing and restful space that supports your body's natural sleep-wake cycle. So take the time to create the perfect sleep environment, and reap the benefits of a restful and rejuvenating night's sleep.

Chapter 12: The Connection Between Sleep and Mental Health

Sleep and mental health are deeply intertwined. It is not uncommon for individuals with mental health disorders to also experience sleep disturbances. At the same time, inadequate or poor-quality sleep can contribute to the development of mental health issues. This chapter will explore the complex relationship between sleep and mental health, including the latest clinical studies and theories, and practical tips for improving sleep and mental health.

The Link Between Sleep and Mental
Health

The relationship between sleep and
mental health is bidirectional. While
mental health disorders can cause sleep
problems, lack of sleep can also contribute
to the development of mental health
issues. In fact, research has shown that
individuals who experience chronic sleep
problems are at a higher risk of developing
mental health disorders.

Sleep disturbances have been linked to a
variety of mental health disorders,
including anxiety, depression, bipolar
disorder, and schizophrenia. For example,

individuals with depression often experience difficulty falling asleep, early morning awakenings, and overall poor sleep quality. Similarly, those with anxiety disorders may struggle with falling asleep due to racing thoughts or have frequent nightmares.

The impact of sleep deprivation on mental health is not limited to adults. A study conducted by the American Psychological Association found that teenagers who experienced insufficient sleep were more likely to experience symptoms of anxiety and depression than those who got adequate sleep.

Theories on the Relationship Between Sleep and Mental Health

While the link between sleep and mental health is well-established, the exact mechanisms behind this relationship are not fully understood. However, several theories have been proposed to explain the connection.

One theory suggests that poor sleep can negatively impact brain function, which can lead to the development of mental health issues. Sleep is essential for the brain to consolidate memories and regulate emotions. When sleep is disrupted, these functions are impaired, which can lead to problems such as depression and anxiety.

Another theory suggests that mental health disorders and sleep disturbances share common underlying mechanisms. For example, both depression and sleep disturbances have been linked to imbalances in neurotransmitters, such as serotonin and dopamine.

Practical Tips for Improving Sleep and Mental Health

1.Improving sleep quality and duration can have a positive impact on mental health.

Here are some practical tips for promoting better sleep and mental health:

2.Stick to a regular sleep schedule: Going to bed and waking up at the same time each day can help regulate your body's internal clock and improve sleep quality.

3.Create a relaxing bedtime routine: Engaging in relaxing activities before bed, such as reading or taking a warm bath, can help prepare your body for sleep.

4.Practice good sleep hygiene: Keep your bedroom cool, dark, and quiet, and avoid using electronic devices in bed.

5.Exercise regularly: Regular physical activity has been shown to improve sleep quality and reduce symptoms of anxiety and depression.

6.Seek treatment for sleep disorders: If you are experiencing chronic sleep problems, consider seeking medical help to address any underlying sleep disorders.

7.Address underlying mental health issues: If you are struggling with mental health issues, seek help from a mental health professional.

Sleep and mental health are closely linked, and inadequate sleep can contribute to the development of mental health disorders. By understanding the connection between sleep and mental health, and implementing practical tips for improving both, individuals can promote better sleep and mental health.

Chapter 13: Sleep and Aging

As we age, our sleep patterns change. We may find ourselves waking up earlier, having trouble falling asleep, or experiencing more sleep disturbances throughout the night. These changes can be frustrating, but they're a normal part of the aging process. In this chapter, we'll explore the connections between sleep and aging, including the ways that aging affects our sleep, the risks associated with sleep problems in older adults, and strategies for promoting healthy sleep as we age.

How Aging Affects Sleep

As we age, our sleep patterns change in a number of ways. Older adults tend to experience less deep sleep and more light sleep than younger adults. They may also spend less time in REM sleep, the stage of sleep when we dream. Additionally, older adults may find it harder to fall asleep and may wake up more often during the night.

These changes are a result of several factors, including changes in our bodies, medications we may be taking, and other health conditions. For example, as we age, our bodies produce less melatonin, the hormone that helps regulate our sleep-wake cycle. This can make it harder to fall asleep and stay asleep.

Medications can also play a role in sleep changes. Many medications commonly taken by older adults, such as diuretics, antidepressants, and beta-blockers, can disrupt sleep. Other health conditions, such as chronic pain, restless leg syndrome, and sleep apnea, can also cause sleep disturbances.

Risks Associated with Sleep Problems in Older Adults

Sleep problems in older adults can have serious consequences. Older adults who don't get enough sleep or who experience poor quality sleep are at higher risk for a range of health problems, including depression, anxiety, and cognitive decline. They're also at higher risk for falls and other accidents, as well as for developing chronic health conditions such as diabetes, heart disease, and obesity.

Strategies for Promoting Healthy Sleep as We Age

While changes in sleep patterns are a natural part of the aging process, there are steps we can take to promote healthy sleep as we age. Here are some strategies to try:

Stick to a regular sleep schedule. Try to go to bed and wake up at the same time each day, even on weekends.

Create a relaxing sleep environment. Make sure your bedroom is cool, quiet, and dark. Consider using blackout curtains, earplugs, or a white noise machine to block out any distractions.

Get regular exercise. Exercise can improve sleep quality and help us fall asleep more easily. Aim for at least 30 minutes of moderate exercise each day, but be sure to finish your workout several hours before bedtime.

Limit caffeine and alcohol. Caffeine and alcohol can both disrupt sleep, so try to avoid them in the hours leading up to bedtime.

Address underlying health issues. If you're experiencing sleep disturbances, talk to your healthcare provider about any underlying health issues that may be contributing to the problem. They may be able to adjust your medications or recommend other treatments to help you sleep better.

Consider natural remedies. Some natural remedies, such as valerian root or chamomile tea, may help promote healthy sleep. Talk to your healthcare provider before trying any new remedies or supplements.

While changes in sleep patterns are a normal part of the aging process, sleep disturbances can have serious consequences for older adults. By taking steps to promote healthy sleep, we can help reduce the risks associated with sleep problems in later life. From creating a relaxing sleep environment to addressing underlying health issues, there are many strategies we can use to improve our sleep as we age.

Chapter 14: Sleep and Children

Sleep is essential for all human beings, but for children, it is even more important. Children require more sleep than adults because their bodies are still developing, and their brains need more time to rest and consolidate information. Lack of adequate sleep can lead to numerous problems for children, including developmental delays, behavioral issues, and even long-term health problems. In this chapter, we will explore the importance of sleep for children, the various factors that affect their sleep patterns, and practical tips for parents to help their children get the sleep they need.

The Importance of Sleep for Children

Sleep plays a critical role in the physical and mental development of children. During sleep, the body produces growth hormones that are essential for children's growth and development. Sleep also plays a crucial role in brain development, especially in young children. During sleep, the brain consolidates the information it has acquired during the day and stores it in long-term memory. This process is essential for learning and cognitive development.

Lack of sleep in children can have significant negative effects. It can affect their behavior, emotional regulation, attention, and academic performance. Inadequate sleep has also been linked to various health problems in children, including obesity, diabetes, and hypertension.

Factors Affecting Children's Sleep

Several factors can affect children's sleep patterns, including age, temperament, sleep environment, and lifestyle. Let's take a closer look at each of these factors.

Age: As children grow and develop, their sleep needs change. Infants need about 14-17 hours of sleep per day, while toddlers need 11-14 hours. Preschoolers require about 10-13 hours of sleep per day, while school-aged children need 9-11 hours of sleep. Teenagers require around 8-10 hours of sleep per day.

Temperament: Some children are naturally better sleepers than others. Children who are more irritable or have more intense emotions may have more difficulty falling asleep and staying asleep.

Sleep environment: A child's sleep environment plays a significant role in their sleep quality. Factors such as noise, light, temperature, and comfort can all affect a child's ability to sleep.

Lifestyle: Children who are active and engage in physical activities during the day tend to sleep better at night. Conversely, children who spend a lot of time in front of screens or have irregular sleep schedules may have difficulty falling asleep.

Practical Tips for Parents

Parents can take several steps to help their children get the sleep they need. Here are some practical tips to consider:

Establish a consistent bedtime routine: Consistency is key to good sleep. Establish a consistent bedtime routine that includes activities such as reading, bath time, or a relaxing bedtime story.

Create a sleep-conducive environment: A quiet, cool, and dark sleep environment can help children fall asleep faster and stay asleep longer.

Encourage physical activity: Encourage your child to engage in physical activities during the day, which can help them sleep better at night.

Limit screen time: Avoid exposing children to screens for at least an hour before bedtime, as the blue light emitted by screens can disrupt sleep.

Monitor your child's diet: Avoid giving your child large meals close to bedtime and limit their intake of sugary or caffeinated foods and drinks.

Seek medical advice if necessary: If you suspect that your child's sleep problems are due to a medical condition, consult your pediatrician.

Sleep is essential for children's physical and mental development. Inadequate sleep can have a significant impact on children's behavior, emotions, academic performance, and long-term health. As parents, it is crucial to prioritize our children's sleep needs and take practical steps to help them get the sleep they need.

Chapter 15: Sleep and Pregnancy

During pregnancy, a woman's body undergoes significant changes that can affect sleep quality and quantity. The most common sleep problems during pregnancy include frequent nighttime urination, heartburn, leg cramps, and insomnia. These issues can occur at any time during pregnancy but are most common in the first and third trimesters. In this chapter, we will discuss the connection between sleep and pregnancy and provide tips for expecting mothers to improve their sleep quality.

The Connection Between Sleep and Pregnancy

Pregnancy causes significant changes in a woman's body, including increased hormone levels, weight gain, and changes in the circulatory and respiratory systems. These changes can result in a variety of sleep disturbances, including:

Insomnia: Insomnia is the most common sleep disorder during pregnancy. Studies suggest that between 50-80% of pregnant women experience insomnia at some point during their pregnancy. This can be due to a variety of factors, including anxiety about the pregnancy, physical discomfort, and hormonal changes.

Restless Leg Syndrome: Restless Leg Syndrome (RLS) is a neurological condition that causes an irresistible urge to move the legs, often accompanied by uncomfortable sensations. RLS can be particularly problematic during pregnancy and is associated with sleep disturbances.

Sleep-Disordered Breathing: Sleep-Disordered Breathing (SDB) includes a range of conditions, such as snoring, sleep apnea, and hypoventilation. SDB is associated with adverse outcomes during pregnancy, including hypertension, gestational diabetes, and preterm delivery.

Periodic Limb Movement Disorder: Periodic Limb Movement Disorder (PLMD) is a sleep disorder characterized by repetitive movements of the legs during sleep. Pregnant women are at higher risk of developing PLMD due to changes in the circulatory system and hormonal changes.

Tips for Improving Sleep Quality During Pregnancy

Establish a consistent sleep schedule: Going to bed and waking up at the same time every day can help regulate the circadian rhythm and improve sleep quality.

Create a relaxing sleep environment: A comfortable mattress, pillows, and bedding can help support the body and reduce physical discomfort. The bedroom should be cool, quiet, and dark to promote relaxation and restful sleep.

Practice relaxation techniques: Relaxation techniques, such as deep breathing, progressive muscle relaxation, and guided imagery, can help reduce stress and promote sleep.

Stay active: Regular exercise during pregnancy can help improve sleep quality and reduce the risk of sleep disturbances. However, pregnant women should consult their healthcare provider before starting or continuing an exercise routine.

Limit caffeine and alcohol intake: Caffeine and alcohol can interfere with sleep quality and should be limited during pregnancy.

Address sleep disorders: Pregnant women with sleep disorders, such as sleep apnea or restless leg syndrome, should discuss treatment options with their healthcare provider.

Sleep is crucial for both the mother and the developing fetus during pregnancy. However, pregnancy can cause significant sleep disturbances that can affect the quality and quantity of sleep. By establishing a consistent sleep schedule, creating a relaxing sleep environment, practicing relaxation techniques, staying active, and addressing sleep disorders, pregnant women can improve their sleep quality and promote overall health and well-being. It is essential for expectant mothers to prioritize their sleep during pregnancy to ensure a healthy and successful pregnancy.

Chapter 16: Sleep and Shift Work

Shift work is a common practice in many industries, such as healthcare, transportation, and manufacturing. It can have significant effects on sleep, health, and quality of life. Shift workers often experience sleep disturbances, fatigue, and decreased performance, which can increase the risk of accidents and errors. In this chapter, we will discuss the impact of shift work on sleep, the mechanisms involved, and practical strategies to improve sleep and reduce the negative consequences of shift work.

The Impact of Shift Work on Sleep

Shift work involves working outside of the regular daytime hours, typically during the night or early morning. This disrupts the natural circadian rhythm, the body's internal clock that regulates sleep and wakefulness. The circadian rhythm is regulated by a group of cells in the hypothalamus that respond to light and dark signals from the environment. The circadian rhythm regulates various physiological processes, including sleep, hormone secretion, body temperature, and metabolism.

Shift work disrupts the circadian rhythm by altering the timing and duration of exposure to light and dark. This can lead to a mismatch between the body's internal clock and the external environment, which can result in sleep disturbances, fatigue, and decreased performance. Shift workers often struggle to fall asleep, stay asleep, and feel rested after sleep. They also tend to experience more daytime sleepiness, fatigue, and cognitive impairments, such as decreased attention, memory, and reaction time.

The mechanisms involved in the impact of shift work on sleep are complex and involve multiple factors. One of the primary mechanisms is the suppression of melatonin, a hormone that is essential for regulating the sleep-wake cycle. Melatonin is produced by the pineal gland in the brain and is released in response to darkness. It promotes sleep by reducing alertness and lowering body temperature. Exposure to light at night can suppress melatonin secretion, leading to reduced sleep quality and quantity.

Another mechanism is the disruption of the social and environmental cues that regulate sleep. Shift workers often have to sleep during the day, which can be challenging due to noise, light, and social disruptions. This can make it difficult to achieve a restful and uninterrupted sleep. Furthermore, shift workers often have irregular work schedules, which can make it challenging to establish a consistent sleep routine.

Practical Strategies to Improve Sleep for Shift Workers

Shift workers can take several practical strategies to improve their sleep and reduce the negative consequences of shift work. Some of these strategies include:

1.Establish a regular sleep schedule: Even if you work irregular hours, try to establish a consistent sleep schedule. This can help your body adjust to the changes in your sleep-wake cycle.

2.Optimize your sleep environment:

Create a sleep-conducive environment by

reducing noise, light, and distractions.

Consider using blackout curtains,

earplugs, or white noise machines to

create a quiet and dark sleep

environment.

3.Use light to your advantage: Exposure

to bright light can help regulate your

circadian rhythm and improve your

alertness during your shift. Use bright

lights at work and during your commute,

and wear dark glasses on your way home

to reduce exposure to daylight.

4.Be mindful of your diet: Avoid heavy meals, caffeine, and alcohol before bedtime, as these can interfere with your sleep quality. Instead, choose lighter meals and non-caffeinated drinks.

5.Take naps: Short naps of 20-30 minutes can help reduce fatigue and improve alertness during your shift. Try to nap during the first part of your shift, when you are most likely to feel sleepy.

6.Seek medical help: If you are experiencing significant sleep problems or other health issues related to shift work, seek medical help from a qualified professional. They can help you develop a personalized treatment plan to improve your sleep and overall health.

Chapter 17: Sleep and Travel

Travel can be an exciting adventure, but it can also disrupt your sleep patterns and impact your overall health and well-being. Whether you're traveling for business or pleasure, crossing time zones or adjusting to a new sleep environment can make it challenging to get a good night's rest. In this chapter, we'll explore the various factors that affect sleep during travel and provide practical tips for ensuring that you get the sleep you need while on the road.

The Science of Sleep and Travel

Traveling can impact your body's natural sleep-wake cycle, also known as your circadian rhythm. The circadian rhythm is responsible for regulating the body's sleep and wake cycles and is primarily influenced by natural light exposure. When traveling, particularly across time zones, your internal clock may become misaligned, leading to symptoms of jet lag, such as fatigue, insomnia, irritability, and difficulty concentrating.

Studies have shown that people who travel frequently, particularly for work, may experience a variety of health problems related to their sleep, including mood disorders, cardiovascular disease, and even cancer. This is thought to be due to the disruption of the circadian rhythm and the body's inability to adapt to new sleep environments quickly.

Factors That Affect Sleep During Travel

There are several factors that can affect your sleep during travel, including:

1.Jet Lag: As mentioned earlier, traveling across time zones can cause a misalignment in your circadian rhythm, leading to symptoms of jet lag.

2.Noise: Whether you're traveling by car, train, or plane, noise can make it difficult to get a good night's sleep.

3.Light: Exposure to light can impact the body's circadian rhythm and make it challenging to fall asleep or stay asleep, particularly if you're in a new time zone.

4.Temperature: The temperature of your sleep environment can also impact your ability to get a good night's rest. If your hotel room is too hot or too cold, it can make it challenging to fall asleep and stay asleep.

5.Comfort: The comfort of your sleep environment, including the quality of the mattress, pillows, and bedding, can impact your ability to get a good night's rest.

Tips for Better Sleep During Travel

1.Plan ahead: If you're traveling across time zones, try to adjust your sleep schedule before you leave. This can help your body adapt to the new time zone more quickly.

2.Pack appropriately: Consider bringing items that can help you sleep, such as earplugs, an eye mask, or a travel pillow.

3.Stay hydrated: Dehydration can exacerbate the symptoms of jet lag, so it's important to drink plenty of water while traveling.

4.Minimize caffeine and alcohol: Caffeine and alcohol can disrupt your sleep, so try to avoid them, particularly close to bedtime.

5.Adjust your sleep environment: If you're staying in a hotel, try to create a sleep-friendly environment by adjusting the temperature, blocking out light and noise, and ensuring that your bed is comfortable.

6.Practice good sleep hygiene: Stick to a regular sleep schedule, even while traveling, and avoid using electronic devices, such as smartphones or tablets, before bedtime.

Finally, for those who frequently travel for work, it's important to try and schedule time for adequate rest and recovery. This may mean scheduling in downtime between meetings or planning for a few days of rest and relaxation following a trip. It's also important to recognize the potential negative impact that frequent travel can have on both sleep and overall health, and to take steps to mitigate these effects as much as possible.

Overall, while travel can be disruptive to our sleep patterns, there are steps we can take to mitigate its impact. By prioritizing good sleep habits, being mindful of our sleep environment, and planning for adequate rest and recovery, we can help ensure that travel doesn't have to mean sacrificing our sleep.

Chapter 18: Dreams and Creativity

Have you ever woken up with a great idea or feeling inspired after a vivid dream? If so, you're not alone. Throughout history, artists, writers, and musicians have credited their dreams with inspiring their most famous works. From Salvador Dali's surrealistic paintings to Mary Shelley's "Frankenstein," dreams have played a significant role in the creative process.

In this chapter, we'll explore the relationship between dreams and creativity, including how dreams can inspire artistic and literary works, and enhance problem-solving abilities. We'll also discuss techniques for harnessing the creative potential of dreams, including keeping a dream journal, using visualization exercises, and practicing lucid dreaming.

The Connection Between Dreams and Creativity

Studies have shown that dreams can be a valuable source of inspiration for creative individuals. Dreams can provide a unique perspective on problems and offer fresh insights into the creative process. In fact, some of the world's most famous inventors and artists have credited their dreams with inspiring their most significant achievements.

One such example is Paul McCartney, who famously wrote the melody for the song "Yesterday" in a dream. Similarly, the scientist Niels Bohr developed the atomic model of the atom after having a dream in which he saw the structure of the atom.

But how do dreams inspire creativity? Some experts believe that the surreal, often illogical nature of dreams allows the mind to make connections that it might not otherwise make. Dreams can also offer a fresh perspective on problems and help individuals think outside the box.

Techniques for Harnessing the Creative Potential of Dreams

One of the most effective ways to tap into the creative potential of dreams is to keep a dream journal. This involves recording your dreams in detail immediately upon waking. By keeping a dream journal, you can gain insight into your subconscious mind and uncover themes and patterns that might inspire creative works.

Another technique is visualization exercises. This involves imagining a scene or event in your mind's eye before going to sleep. By visualizing the scene, you can create a mental space for your dreams to play out in a specific direction, allowing you to take control of the direction of your dreams and potentially influence their creative output.

Finally, practicing lucid dreaming can be a powerful tool for enhancing creativity. Lucid dreaming is a state in which the dreamer is aware that they are dreaming and can actively participate in the dream. By learning to control their dreams, creative individuals can direct their dreams towards specific creative goals.

In addition, there are several scientific theories about how dreams and creativity are related. One theory is that during REM sleep, the brain is able to make new connections between seemingly unrelated ideas. This can lead to new insights and ideas that can be used in creative work.

Another theory is that dreams are a way for the brain to process complex information and emotions. Dreams can help us make sense of our experiences and emotions in new and unexpected ways. This can lead to new insights and creative ideas.

Dreams have been a significant source of inspiration for artists, writers, and musicians throughout history. They offer a unique perspective on the creative process and can provide fresh insights into problem-solving. By harnessing the creative potential of dreams, individuals can tap into a powerful tool for enhancing their creativity.

Whether through keeping a dream journal, practicing visualization exercises, or developing lucid dreaming skills, anyone can learn to use their dreams to enhance their creative output. By exploring the connection between dreams and creativity and practicing the techniques outlined in this chapter, readers can tap into the full potential of their subconscious mind and unlock new levels of creativity.

Chapter 19: Sleep and Productivity

Sleep and productivity are closely intertwined. Poor sleep quality can negatively impact work performance, creativity, and decision-making abilities, while improving sleep can enhance productivity and job satisfaction. In this chapter, we'll explore the relationship between sleep and productivity, examine the factors that contribute to poor sleep quality, and provide strategies to improve sleep and boost productivity.

The Impact of Sleep on Productivity

A good night's sleep is essential for optimal cognitive and physical functioning. Studies have shown that lack of sleep can impair attention, memory, and problem-solving abilities. Moreover, it can affect mood and lead to decreased job satisfaction and increased absenteeism. This is because when you are tired, it is more difficult to focus and complete tasks efficiently, leading to decreased productivity.

In contrast, adequate sleep has been linked to improved cognitive function, better memory, and increased creativity. Studies have shown that sleep enhances problem-solving abilities, promotes creativity and helps to consolidate newly learned information. Therefore, getting enough sleep can positively affect performance, job satisfaction, and overall quality of life.

Factors Contributing to Poor Sleep Quality

Several factors can contribute to poor sleep quality, including lifestyle factors, such as work and social schedules, and medical conditions. Sleep disorders like insomnia, sleep apnea, and restless leg syndrome can also negatively impact sleep quality.

Working long hours or night shifts can interfere with the natural circadian rhythm, which can lead to sleep problems. Moreover, the increased use of electronic devices before bed can disrupt the production of melatonin, the hormone that regulates sleep. Additionally, high levels of stress and anxiety can affect sleep, making it difficult to fall or stay asleep.

Strategies to Improve Sleep Quality and Boost Productivity

Improving sleep quality can significantly enhance productivity and job satisfaction. Here are some strategies that can help you get a better night's sleep:

Maintain a Regular Sleep Schedule: Going to bed and waking up at the same time each day can help regulate your body's natural circadian rhythm, which can lead to better sleep quality.

Improve Sleep Hygiene: This includes creating a sleep-conducive environment, such as keeping the bedroom cool, dark, and quiet. It also involves limiting screen time before bed, avoiding caffeine and alcohol before sleep, and developing a relaxing bedtime routine.

Address Sleep Problems with Behavioral Interventions: If you have a sleep disorder, cognitive-behavioral therapy (CBT) can help address the underlying issues that contribute to the problem. CBT for insomnia is a widely used approach that focuses on improving sleep hygiene, developing relaxation techniques, and addressing negative sleep-related thoughts.

Implement Mindfulness Techniques: Mindfulness-based practices, such as meditation and deep breathing, can reduce stress and anxiety, and can help promote better sleep. These techniques can be used before bed or during the day to help manage stress levels.

Exercise Regularly: Exercise has been shown to improve sleep quality and promote relaxation. However, it is important to avoid exercising close to bedtime, as it can increase alertness and make it more difficult to fall asleep.

Consider Light Therapy: Light therapy is a technique used to reset the circadian rhythm by exposing the eyes to bright light at specific times of the day. This can be particularly helpful for individuals who work night shifts or have trouble adjusting to time zone changes during travel.

Harnessing the Creative Potential of Dreams

Dreams have long been associated with creativity and problem-solving abilities. Many artists, writers, and scientists have credited their dreams with inspiring their work or providing solutions to complex problems. Dreams can offer unique perspectives and insights that may not be available during waking hours.

Keeping a dream journal can be a helpful tool for harnessing the creative potential of dreams. Recording dreams immediately upon waking can help capture details that may otherwise be forgotten. Visualization exercises can also be useful in promoting creative problem-solving during waking hours. These exercises involve visualizing specific goals or challenges, and then imagining creative solutions.

Lucid dreaming is another technique that can help individuals harness the creative potential of dreams. Lucid dreaming is the act of becoming aware that you are dreaming while still in the dream state. This can provide a unique opportunity to explore and manipulate the dream world, potentially leading to enhanced creativity and problem-solving abilities.

Sleep and productivity are intimately connected, with adequate sleep being essential for optimal cognitive and physical functioning. The factors contributing to poor sleep quality are numerous, ranging from medical conditions to lifestyle factors. Implementing strategies to improve sleep quality, such as maintaining a regular sleep schedule and developing a relaxing bedtime routine, can lead to enhanced productivity and job satisfaction.

Dreams also offer unique potential for creativity and problem-solving. Keeping a dream journal, practicing visualization exercises, and exploring lucid dreaming can all help individuals harness this potential. By prioritizing sleep and tapping into the creative potential of dreams, individuals can enhance their productivity, creativity, and overall quality of life.

Chapter 20: Sleep and Relationships

Sleep is a vital aspect of our physical and mental well-being, and it is essential to our relationships as well. Sleep affects not only our own health but also the way we interact with others, particularly our partners. The quality and quantity of sleep can significantly impact our relationships, and sleep deprivation can cause tension and conflict in even the most loving relationships. This chapter will explore the relationship between sleep and relationships, including the impact of sleep on relationships and strategies to promote healthy sleep habits in relationships.

The Impact of Sleep on Relationships

Sleep plays a crucial role in regulating our emotions and behaviors. When we don't get enough sleep, it can negatively affect our mood, cognition, and decision-making abilities. Poor sleep quality can also lead to irritability, frustration, and decreased empathy. These factors can all contribute to tension and conflict in a relationship.

Sleep deprivation can also have a significant impact on our physical health, which can further strain our relationships. Lack of sleep can lead to weakened immunity, increased susceptibility to illness, and a higher risk of chronic health conditions such as obesity, diabetes, and heart disease. These health problems can cause stress and anxiety, leading to further tension and conflict in relationships.

Additionally, sleep deprivation can negatively affect sexual intimacy and emotional connection in relationships. Sleep-deprived partners are less likely to engage in physical intimacy and have lower sexual desire. This can cause a decrease in emotional intimacy and can create a disconnect between partners.

Strategies to Promote Healthy Sleep Habits in Relationships

There are several strategies couples can use to promote healthy sleep habits in their relationships. These strategies can help to reduce tension and conflict and increase emotional and physical intimacy.

Communicate About Sleep Needs and Preferences

Communication is key to any healthy relationship, and this is no different when it comes to sleep. Couples should discuss their sleep needs and preferences and work together to create a sleep routine that works for both partners. This includes setting a regular bedtime, discussing bedtime routines, and creating a sleep-conducive environment that is comfortable for both partners.

Create a Relaxing Sleep Environment

Creating a relaxing sleep environment is essential to getting a good night's sleep. This includes having a comfortable bed and pillows, keeping the room cool and dark, and minimizing noise and light. Couples can work together to create a sleep-conducive environment that is comfortable for both partners. This may involve using earplugs, white noise machines, or other tools to block out noise.

Address Sleep Problems with Behavioral
Interventions

Behavioral interventions such as
cognitive-behavioral therapy (CBT) can be
effective in addressing sleep problems
such as insomnia. Couples can work
together to identify any sleep problems
they may be experiencing and seek out
professional help if needed. CBT can help
to address negative thoughts and beliefs
about sleep and create a healthier sleep
routine.

Prioritize Sleep Hygiene

Sleep hygiene refers to the practices and habits that promote healthy sleep. Couples can work together to prioritize sleep hygiene by creating a regular sleep routine, avoiding caffeine and alcohol before bedtime, and minimizing screen time before bed. These practices can help to promote healthy sleep and reduce tension and conflict in relationships.

Sleep is an essential component of our physical and mental health, and it also plays a vital role in our relationships. Poor sleep quality can negatively impact our mood, cognition, and decision-making abilities, and can lead to tension and conflict in relationships. Strategies such as communication, creating a relaxing sleep environment, addressing sleep problems with behavioral interventions, and prioritizing sleep hygiene can help to promote healthy sleep habits in relationships. By working together to improve sleep quality, couples can enhance their emotional and physical intimacy and reduce tension and conflict in their relationships.

Chapter 21: Dreams and Spiritual Practices

Throughout history, dreams have played a significant role in various spiritual practices. Many cultures view dreams as a powerful source of guidance, insight, and spiritual connection. This chapter explores the relationship between dreams and spiritual practices and provides unique ideas for integrating dreams into these practices.

The Role of Dreams in Spiritual Practices

Dreams have been an essential part of spiritual practices since ancient times. In

many cultures, dreams are viewed as a
form of communication from the divine,
offering insights and guidance on a
person's spiritual journey. Some of the
earliest known records of dream
interpretation come from ancient Egypt,
where dreams were considered a window
into the realm of the gods.

Similarly, in many indigenous cultures,
dreams are seen as a connection to the
spiritual world. For example, in many
Native American cultures, dreams are
used as a source of wisdom and
guidance. Many Aboriginal cultures in
Australia also place a strong emphasis on
dreams, using them to understand the

spiritual connections between all living beings.

The significance of dreams in spirituality is also evident in major religions. In the Bible, for example, many significant events and messages are conveyed through dreams. In the Old Testament, Joseph's dreams foretold his rise to power, and in the New Testament, an angel appeared in a dream to Joseph, guiding him to take Mary as his wife. Similarly, in the Islamic tradition, the Prophet Muhammad is said to have received revelations in his dreams.

Dreams and Spiritual Growth

One of the essential roles of dreams in spiritual practices is facilitating personal growth and development. Dreams can offer insights into the unconscious mind, revealing patterns of thought and behavior that may be hindering spiritual progress. They can also reveal repressed emotions and desires that need to be acknowledged and integrated into one's spiritual journey.

Dreams can also provide guidance on a person's spiritual path. For example, dreams may offer insight into one's purpose, provide clarity on a particular decision or issue, or offer guidance on how to overcome a spiritual obstacle.

Many spiritual teachers also believe that dreams can facilitate spiritual awakening, leading to a deeper understanding of the self and the world.

Integrating Dreams into Spiritual Practices

There are various techniques for integrating dreams into spiritual practices, allowing individuals to harness the power of their dreams for spiritual growth and development. Some of these techniques include:

Dream Journaling: Keeping a dream journal is one of the most effective ways to connect with and remember dreams. A dream journal allows individuals to record their dreams immediately upon waking, helping to solidify their memory of the dream. Over time, a dream journal can reveal patterns and themes in dreams that may provide valuable insight into one's spiritual journey.

Dream Interpretation: Dream interpretation involves analyzing the symbolism and imagery in dreams to gain insight into their meaning. Many spiritual traditions have developed systems for interpreting dreams, which can provide valuable guidance and insight for individuals.

Dream Incubation: Dream incubation is the practice of focusing on a specific question or issue before going to bed, with the intention of receiving guidance in the form of a dream. This technique involves setting a clear intention before falling asleep and creating a calm and relaxing environment conducive to dreaming.

Lucid Dreaming: Lucid dreaming is the ability to become aware that one is dreaming while in the dream state. This awareness allows individuals to consciously control their dreams, using them to explore and resolve spiritual issues or gain insights into their spiritual journey.

There are many benefits to using dreams in spiritual practices, including:

Gaining insight and guidance: Dreams can offer valuable insights and guidance for spiritual growth and personal development. By exploring the symbolism and meaning behind our dreams, we can gain a deeper understanding of ourselves and our path.

Promoting healing and transformation: Dreams can help us identify unresolved issues and patterns in our lives, and bring them to the surface for healing and transformation.

Connecting with a higher power: Dreams can provide a sense of connection with a higher power or a divine source. By receiving messages and guidance in our dreams, we can feel supported and guided on our spiritual path.

Enhancing creativity: Dreams can be a rich source of inspiration for artistic and creative works. By tapping into the creative potential of our dreams, we can enhance our artistic abilities and bring new ideas to life.

Overall, dreams have played a significant role in spiritual practices throughout history. By exploring the symbolism and meaning behind our dreams, we can gain valuable insights and guidance for spiritual growth and personal development. Techniques such as dream incubation, dream interpretation, and lucid dreaming can be used to integrate dreams into spiritual practices. The benefits of using dreams in spiritual practices include gaining insight and guidance, promoting healing and transformation, connecting with a higher power, and enhancing creativity.

Chapter 22: How to Create a Sleep Routine

Having a consistent sleep routine is one of the most effective ways to improve the quality and quantity of your sleep. In this chapter, we'll explore the importance of a sleep routine, steps to create one, and strategies to stick to it.

The Importance of a Sleep Routine

Your body thrives on routine, and your sleep is no exception. When you establish a regular sleep routine, your body learns to anticipate and prepare for sleep, making it easier to fall asleep and stay asleep throughout the night.

A sleep routine can also help regulate your body's internal clock, known as the circadian rhythm. This clock regulates many of your body's functions, including sleep-wake cycles, hunger, and hormones. By sticking to a consistent sleep routine, you help train your body to naturally follow this rhythm, leading to better overall health.

Creating a Sleep Routine

Creating a sleep routine can seem daunting, but it doesn't have to be complicated. Here are some steps to follow when creating a sleep routine:

Set a Consistent Bedtime and Wake-Up Time

The first step to creating a sleep routine is to establish a consistent bedtime and wake-up time. Aim to go to bed and wake up at the same time every day, including on weekends. This consistency will help regulate your body's internal clock and make it easier to fall asleep and wake up each day.

Wind Down Before Bed

Create a relaxing bedtime routine that helps you wind down and prepare for sleep. This could include taking a warm bath or shower, reading a book, or practicing meditation or deep breathing exercises. Avoid stimulating activities before bed, such as watching TV or using electronic devices, as they can disrupt your sleep.

Create a Sleep-Conducive Environment

Your sleep environment can greatly impact the quality of your sleep. Create a sleep-conducive environment by keeping your bedroom cool, quiet, and dark. Consider investing in blackout curtains, earplugs, or a white noise machine to help create an optimal sleep environment.

Limit Caffeine and Alcohol

Caffeine and alcohol can greatly impact the quality of your sleep. Avoid consuming these substances before bed, as they can interfere with your ability to fall asleep and stay asleep throughout the night.

Get Regular Exercise

Regular exercise can help regulate your body's internal clock and improve the quality of your sleep. Aim to get at least 30 minutes of moderate exercise each day, such as walking, biking, or swimming. Just be sure to avoid exercising too close to bedtime, as it can interfere with your ability to fall asleep.

Sticking to a Sleep Routine

Once you have established your sleep routine, it is essential to stick to it. Here are some strategies that can help you maintain your sleep routine:

Set a consistent bedtime and wake-up time: Going to bed and waking up at the same time every day can help regulate your body's internal clock and make it easier to fall asleep and wake up naturally.

Avoid electronics before bedtime: The blue light emitted by electronic devices can suppress the production of melatonin, making it harder to fall asleep. Avoid using electronic devices at least an hour before bedtime.

Make your bedroom conducive to sleep: Keep your bedroom cool, dark, and quiet, and use comfortable bedding and pillows to create a relaxing sleep environment.

Limit caffeine and alcohol consumption: Caffeine and alcohol can interfere with sleep quality and should be consumed in moderation, especially before bedtime.

Stick to your routine on weekends: It can be tempting to stay up late and sleep in on the weekends, but this can disrupt your sleep routine. Try to stick to your routine as much as possible on weekends.

Use relaxation techniques: If you have trouble falling asleep, try relaxation techniques such as deep breathing, progressive muscle relaxation, or visualization to calm your mind and body.

Address sleep problems promptly: If you experience persistent sleep problems despite following a sleep routine, it is important to seek professional help to identify and address any underlying sleep disorders or medical conditions.

Creating a sleep routine can be a highly effective way to improve the quality and quantity of your sleep, leading to numerous benefits for your physical and mental health. By following the steps outlined in this chapter, you can create a sleep routine that works for you and learn strategies to stick to it for long-term success.

Remember, improving your sleep habits requires patience, persistence, and a willingness to make changes to your lifestyle. With the right mindset and a commitment to your sleep routine, you can enjoy the benefits of better sleep and wake up feeling refreshed and energized each day.

Chapter 23: The Benefits of Napping

For some people, napping is seen as a sign of laziness or lack of productivity. However, research shows that taking a nap can actually have numerous benefits for both physical and mental health. In this chapter, we'll explore the benefits of napping and how to make the most of your nap time.

The Benefits of Napping:

1.Boosts Cognitive Function: Napping has been shown to enhance cognitive function, including memory, creativity, and problem-solving abilities. A study conducted by NASA on military pilots and astronauts found that a 40-minute nap improved their cognitive performance by 35% and alertness by 100%. This increase in cognitive function is attributed to the brain's ability to consolidate memories and processes during sleep.

2.Improves Physical Health: Napping can also have positive effects on physical health. A study published in the Journal of Clinical Endocrinology & Metabolism found that a 30-minute nap improved insulin sensitivity, which can reduce the risk of type 2 diabetes. Additionally, napping has been linked to lower blood pressure, reduced stress, and improved immune system function.

3.Increases Alertness: Napping can help combat daytime sleepiness and increase alertness. This is particularly useful for people who work long hours, work late at night, or have interrupted sleep schedules. A short nap of 20-30 minutes has been shown to significantly increase alertness and reduce sleepiness.

4.Enhances Mood: Napping can also have positive effects on mood. Studies have found that a nap can improve mood and reduce feelings of fatigue and irritability.

This is particularly true for people who are sleep deprived or have insomnia.

Steps to Take a Nap:

1.Determine the Best Time: The ideal time to nap is in the early afternoon, around 1-3 pm, when the body's natural circadian rhythm dips. This is when most people experience a natural slump in energy and alertness.

2.Set the Scene: The environment in which you nap is important. Make sure the room is cool, dark, and quiet. Use earplugs or a white noise machine to block out any distracting sounds. Also,

make sure to set an alarm to avoid
oversleeping and disrupting your
nighttime sleep.

3.Keep it Short: The ideal nap should be
no longer than 30 minutes. Longer naps
can lead to grogginess and interfere with
nighttime sleep. A short nap of 10-20
minutes can be enough to boost
alertness and cognitive function without
causing drowsiness.

4.Nap Consistently: Consistency is key
when it comes to napping. Try to take a
nap at the same time every day to train
your body to relax and sleep during this
time.

5.Listen to Your Body: Finally, it's important to listen to your body and be aware of your individual sleep needs. If you feel tired or sleepy, take a nap. If you're feeling energized and alert, skip the nap.

Strategies to Make the Most of Your Nap Time:

1.Power Nap: A power nap is a short nap of 10-20 minutes designed to provide a quick burst of energy and alertness. This type of nap is ideal for people who need a quick boost of energy to get through the day.

2.Nap for Memory Consolidation: If you need to remember something important, taking a nap after learning it can help consolidate the memory. This is because the brain processes and stores information during sleep.

3.Use a Coffee Nap: A coffee nap is a technique in which you drink a cup of coffee before taking a short nap. The caffeine takes about 20-30 minutes to kick in, which is the ideal amount of time for a power nap.

Overall, napping can be a helpful tool for improving cognitive function, productivity, and overall well-being. By following these best practices, individuals can reap the benefits of napping while avoiding potential downsides.

Chapter 24: Dreams and Therapy

Dreams have been a subject of fascination for humans for thousands of years. They are often seen as a window into the subconscious mind and can provide insight into one's emotional and mental state. For this reason, dreams have been used in therapy as a tool to facilitate personal growth and healing. In this chapter, we will explore the relationship between dreams and therapy, and the benefits of using dreams in the therapeutic process.

Dreams in Therapy

Dreams have been used in therapy for centuries, dating back to ancient civilizations such as the Greeks and Egyptians. In modern times, dream analysis was popularized by the work of Sigmund Freud, who believed that dreams were a way for the unconscious mind to communicate with the conscious mind. Freud developed a method of dream analysis called psychoanalysis, which involves exploring the symbols and themes present in dreams to uncover the hidden meanings and messages behind them.

While psychoanalysis is still used today, other forms of therapy have also incorporated dreams as a tool for personal growth and healing. Jungian therapy, developed by Carl Jung, emphasizes the importance of dreams as a source of insight into the unconscious mind. In Jungian therapy, dreams are seen as a way for the individual to communicate with their psyche, and the therapist works with the client to explore the symbolism and themes present in their dreams.

Benefits of Using Dreams in Therapy

There are many benefits to using dreams in therapy. Dreams can provide insight into one's emotional and mental state, and can highlight underlying issues that may be affecting one's well-being. Through exploring dreams, individuals can gain a better understanding of themselves and their experiences, and can work towards resolving issues that may be impacting their mental health.

Dreams can also be used to facilitate personal growth and self-discovery. By exploring the themes and symbols present in their dreams, individuals can gain a deeper understanding of their values, beliefs, and desires. This can lead to increased self-awareness and a greater sense of purpose in life.

Additionally, dreams can be used to address specific issues that may be affecting one's mental health. For example, recurring nightmares may be a symptom of post-traumatic stress disorder, and exploring these nightmares in therapy can help individuals process their trauma and develop coping strategies.

Using Dreams in Therapy

Incorporating dreams into therapy can take many forms. One common method is dream journaling, where individuals write down their dreams upon waking and then explore the themes and symbols present in the dream. This can be done on one's own, or with the guidance of a therapist. Another method is to use visualization exercises to explore a dream in greater detail. This can involve recreating the dream in one's mind and exploring the symbolism and themes in a safe and controlled environment.

Lucid dreaming is another technique that can be used in therapy. Lucid dreaming is when an individual becomes aware that they are dreaming and can then control the dream. This can be a powerful tool for individuals to work through issues in a safe and controlled environment.

It is important to note that while dreams can be a useful tool in therapy, they should not be used as the sole method of treatment. Dreams should be explored in conjunction with other therapeutic techniques, and individuals should work with a trained therapist to ensure that they are being used in a safe and effective manner.

Dreams have been used in therapy for centuries, and for good reason. They can provide insight into one's emotional and mental state, facilitate personal growth and self-discovery, and be used to address specific issues that may be impacting one's mental health. By exploring dreams in therapy, individuals can gain a better understanding of themselves and their experiences, and work towards resolving underlying issues.

Chapter 25: How to Overcome Insomnia

Insomnia is a common sleep disorder that affects millions of people worldwide. It can be caused by various factors, including stress, anxiety, depression, medical conditions, and certain medications. Insomnia can disrupt your daily life, affecting your mood, productivity, and overall health. Fortunately, there are effective strategies to overcome insomnia and improve the quality of your sleep.

Step 1: Identify the underlying cause

The first step in overcoming insomnia is to identify the underlying cause of your sleep disturbance. This can involve an assessment of your sleep patterns, medical history, and current lifestyle habits. Common causes of insomnia include stress, anxiety, depression, chronic pain, caffeine or alcohol consumption, and medication use. Once the underlying cause has been identified, the appropriate treatment can be implemented.

Step 2: Adopt healthy sleep habits

In addition to addressing the underlying cause of your insomnia, adopting healthy sleep habits can improve your chances of getting a good night's sleep. Some of the recommended sleep habits include:

1.Maintaining a regular sleep schedule: Go to bed and wake up at the same time every day, even on weekends.

2.Creating a sleep-conducive environment: Keep your bedroom dark, cool, and quiet. Use comfortable bedding and avoid watching TV or using electronic devices in bed.

3.Avoiding stimulating activities before bedtime: Avoid engaging in activities that can cause excitement or stress, such as working or exercising, right before bedtime.

4.Avoiding caffeine, nicotine, and alcohol:

These substances can interfere with

sleep and should be avoided, especially

close to bedtime.

5.Practicing relaxation techniques:

Techniques such as deep breathing,

meditation, or yoga can help you relax

and prepare for sleep.

Step 3: Cognitive-behavioral therapy for

insomnia (CBT-I)

Cognitive-behavioral therapy for insomnia

(CBT-I) is a highly effective treatment for

chronic insomnia. CBT-I is a type of talk

therapy that focuses on changing the

negative thoughts and behaviors that are

associated with insomnia. CBT-I typically involves several components, including sleep hygiene education, stimulus control, sleep restriction, and cognitive therapy.

Sleep hygiene education: This component of CBT-I involves teaching patients about the importance of good sleep hygiene and the factors that can interfere with sleep.

Stimulus control: This involves creating an association between the bedroom and sleep, and removing factors that can interfere with sleep. For example, patients may be advised to avoid doing non-sleep activities in the bedroom, such as working or watching TV.

Sleep restriction: This involves limiting the amount of time spent in bed to increase the amount of time spent asleep. For example, patients may be advised to only spend six hours in bed, even if they have trouble falling asleep at first. As sleep efficiency improves, the time in bed can gradually be increased.

Cognitive therapy: This component of CBT-I involves identifying and changing negative thoughts and beliefs about sleep. Patients may be encouraged to reframe their thoughts and beliefs about sleep and develop more positive associations with sleep.

Step 4: Medication

Medication can be used to treat insomnia in some cases. However, medication should be used cautiously and only under the guidance of a healthcare professional. There are several classes of medication that can be used to treat insomnia, including benzodiazepines, nonbenzodiazepines, and melatonin agonists. These medications can have side effects and should only be used as a short-term solution.

Step 5: Address underlying medical conditions

In some cases, insomnia may be caused by an underlying medical condition. For example, sleep apnea, restless leg syndrome, and other sleep disorders can cause insomnia. Treating the underlying medical condition can often improve sleep quality.

Insomnia can be a frustrating and debilitating condition, but there are effective strategies to overcome it. By addressing underlying issues, creating a sleep-conducive environment, and developing healthy sleep habits, it is possible to achieve restful and restorative sleep.

Chapter 26: Sleep and Dreams in the Post-COVID World

The COVID-19 pandemic has had a significant impact on every aspect of life, including sleep and dreams. From disrupted routines to increased anxiety, the pandemic has affected how we sleep and the content of our dreams. As we are moving into a post-COVID world, it is essential to understand the implications of these changes and how to adapt to them.

The Effects of COVID-19 on Sleep

The pandemic has had a significant impact on sleep patterns. With many people working from home or out of work entirely, the boundaries between work and home life have become blurred, leading to a breakdown of routines. Increased stress and anxiety have also contributed to poor sleep quality, with many people reporting difficulty falling asleep or staying asleep.

Studies have shown that the pandemic has led to an increase in insomnia and other sleep disorders. In a survey conducted by the American Academy of Sleep Medicine, 56% of respondents reported having difficulty sleeping during the pandemic, while 19% reported a new onset of insomnia.

The Effects of COVID-19 on Dreams

The pandemic has also had an impact on the content of our dreams. Many people have reported having more vivid and emotional dreams, with themes of stress, anxiety, and uncertainty. A study published in the Journal of Sleep Research found that 29% of participants reported an increase in pandemic-related dreams, with themes of illness, death, and social distancing.

Some experts believe that the increase in vivid and emotional dreams is due to the increased stress and anxiety caused by the pandemic. Dreams are the brain's way of processing emotions and experiences, so it is not surprising that the content of our dreams reflects our current state of mind.

How to Adapt to Changes in Sleep and Dreams

As we are moving into a post-COVID world, it is important to understand how the pandemic has affected our sleep and dreams and to take steps to adapt to these changes.

Stick to a Routine: Establishing a regular sleep routine can help improve sleep quality and reduce insomnia. Set a regular bedtime and wake-up time, and try to stick to this schedule as much as possible.

Practice Good Sleep Hygiene: Practice good sleep hygiene by creating a comfortable sleep environment, avoiding stimulants like caffeine and electronics before bed, and engaging in relaxing activities before sleep.

Manage Stress and Anxiety: Stress and anxiety are common during times of uncertainty, but there are ways to manage these feelings. Engage in stress-reducing activities like meditation or yoga, and consider talking to a mental health professional if you are experiencing significant stress or anxiety.

Journal Your Dreams: Keeping a dream journal can help you process and understand the content of your dreams. Write down the details of your dreams as soon as you wake up, and look for patterns or recurring themes.

Practice Lucid Dreaming: Lucid dreaming is the practice of becoming aware that you are dreaming and taking control of the dream's content. This practice can help you process emotions and overcome fears in a safe and controlled environment.

The COVID-19 pandemic has had a significant impact on sleep and dreams, with many people experiencing disrupted sleep patterns and increased vivid and emotional dreams. As we are moving into a post-COVID world, it is important to understand these changes and take steps to adapt to them. By practicing good sleep hygiene, managing stress and anxiety, and exploring techniques like lucid dreaming, we can improve our sleep and use our dreams as a tool for personal growth and healing.

Chapter 27: The Future of Sleep and Dream Science

As we continue to learn more about sleep and dreams, the future of sleep and dream science holds great promise. Here are some of the exciting directions in which sleep and dream science is heading.

The role of genetics: As genetic research continues to advance, we may gain a better understanding of how our genes influence our sleep and dreaming patterns. This could lead to personalized treatments for sleep disorders and more targeted approaches to improving sleep quality.

The use of technology: Advances in technology are allowing for more sophisticated monitoring and analysis of sleep patterns. This includes wearable devices that can track sleep stages and detect sleep disturbances, as well as apps that can provide personalized sleep recommendations and track sleep improvement over time.

Integrating sleep and mental health treatment: As we continue to learn more about the connection between sleep and mental health, we may see more integration of sleep treatment with mental health treatment. This could involve incorporating cognitive-behavioral therapy for insomnia into mental health treatment plans, or developing treatments for sleep disorders that are tailored to individuals with specific mental health conditions.

The study of dreams: As we gain a better understanding of the neuroscience of dreams, we may see more research on the function of dreams and how they relate to memory consolidation, problem-solving, and emotional processing. This could lead to new approaches for using dreams to enhance learning, creativity, and emotional well-being.

The impact of environmental factors: As our understanding of the impact of environmental factors on sleep continues to grow, we may see more efforts to create sleep-friendly environments in workplaces, schools, and public spaces. This could include innovations in lighting, temperature control, and noise reduction, as well as changes in social norms around sleep and work.

In conclusion, the future of sleep and dream science holds great promise for improving our understanding of these essential aspects of human health and well-being. As we continue to uncover new insights and develop new tools for understanding and enhancing sleep and dreaming, we can look forward to a future in which we all sleep better and dream more deeply.

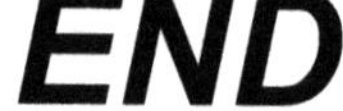

END

www.ingramcontent.com/pod-product-compliance
Lightning Source LLC
Chambersburg PA
CBHW061602250726
48657CB00017B/1243